How to Get Pregnant, Expecting Fast:

Getting Pregnant Fertility Herbs, Exercises, Diet Guide

By

Eva Delano

Table of Contents

Introduction 5

Chapter 1. Tips You Can Do to Get Pregnant 7

Chapter 2. Pregnancy Exercises 14

Chapter 3. Diet Guidelines For Pregnant Women 16

Chapter 4. Herbs That Can Help You Get Pregnant 18

Chapter 5. When to Test For Pregnancy 20

Chapter 6. How Age Affects Pregnancy 21

Chapter 7. How to Find Out if You Are Ovulating 23

Chapter 8. How to Deal With a Miscarriage 25

Conclusion 27

Thank You Page 29

How to Get Pregnant, Expecting Fast: Getting Pregnant Fertility Herbs, Exercises, Diet Guide

By Eva Delano

© Copyright 2015 Eva Delano

Reproduction or translation of any part of this work beyond that permitted by section 107 or 108 of the 1976 United States Copyright Act without permission of the copyright owner is unlawful. Requests for permission or further information should be addressed to the author.

This publication is designed to provide accurate and authoritative information in regard to the subject matter covered. This work is sold with the understanding that the publisher is not engaged in rendering legal, accounting, or other professional services. If legal advice or other expert assistance is required, the services of a competent professional person should be sought.

First Published, 2015

Printed in the United States of America

Introduction

There are couples today who try for years to have a baby, but have not been very successful or they end up consuming too much time. This can cause them to have just one child instead of 2 or 3 which is what they really wanted. This is because a woman can only conceive up to a certain age and anytime beyond that could be a threat to their lives. This is another reason why couples cannot consume too much time trying to get pregnant and they should be aware, especially the woman, on what are the things that need to be done in order to have a baby exactly at the time that they have planned.

This book will give you tips on how to get pregnant, what exercises you need to do to get pregnant, what kind of diet you need to have, if there are herbs you can take to help you get pregnant, when you should test for pregnancy, how age affects pregnancy, how you will know if you are ovulating, and how to deal with a miscarriage in case you go through one. Getting pregnant is a beautiful thing and there is nothing more that couples would want so after you have read this book, you will be able to apply these things in your life to have a better chance at getting pregnant. You will also be able to figure out what you have been doing wrong or what are the things you need to change about your diet, exercise, lifestyle or in general. Knowing what you can do to become successful in your efforts will help you and your husband figure out what you can do as a couple too. If you are experiencing stressors in your life, you should also be able to overcome them because being stressed can also prevent pregnancy and this was mentioned because stress has become a natural part of human lives. You might think that something as simple as stress does not have anything to do with why you are not getting pregnant, but the reality is stress affects your overall condition and you need to be healthy enough to get pregnant.

Finish reading this book so that you will have the proper knowledge about how you can get pregnant.

Chapter 1. Tips You Can Do to Get Pregnant

You need to frequently record your menstrual cycle because if you want to have a baby, you should be able to monitor if your period's first days come regularly each month. This means that if the first days of your period come every month with the same number of days between them. There are women who have an irregular period which means that the cycle of your menstruation can vary every month. If you are able to track this down using a calendar, you will have a better chance of getting pregnant because you will know when you are ovulating. The egg of a woman is only fertile for 12 to 24 hours after it has been released, but the sperm of a man can live inside a woman's body for up to 6 days. You should also monitor the time when you are ovulating because if you have a regular menstrual cycle, this means that you are ovulating 2 weeks before the day of your period. Those women who are experiencing irregular cycle have a harder time knowing when they are ovulating, but usually it happens 12 to 16 days prior to the start of their next period. You can buy ovulation-prediction kits because it can help predict if the woman is ovulating. You just need to follow the instructions well so that you will be able to safely use it. There are kits sold in drug stores which test your urine for luteinizing hormone which is a substance that increases its levels every month at the time of the ovulation and this will be the reason for the ovaries to release an egg. When you get a positive result, you must have sex 3 days after because this is when you will be able to increase your chances of getting pregnant. Another way to tell if a woman is ovulating is to do the basal body temperature method this is by taking the body temperature every morning and put it on a chart using a graph and monitor this for not less than 3 menstrual cycles. Right after ovulation, the body temperature of a woman increases by less than half a degree which usually 0.3 Celsius degrees. The first 2 to 3 days before the temperature rises are the days when the woman is most fertile. Another way to check is if you have mucus in the vagina because it means that you have 2.3 times higher chance of becoming pregnant in the next 6 months. Before the ovulation occurs, the amount of the mucus will increase right before the ovulation and there is an increase in the amount of the mucus. The mucus also becomes more and slippery which means that the woman is most fertile. When the mucus in the cervix becomes slipper, the sperm will have an easier time to make it into the egg. When you already know your fertility window, have sex every other day because the fertile window happens with a 5-day interval before the ovulation and during ovulation. These are the woman's most fertile days. Intercourse gets your successfully pregnant if you do it 2 days before you ovulate. There is a research which shows that having sex every day during the fertility window makes no significance difference to those have sex every other day. Having sex every other day might be something that couples find easier to do. You should also have a healthy body weight when trying to conceive because of you are too heavy, it can decrease your chances of getting pregnant, but if you are too thin, you will also have a hard time having a baby. There is a research showing that a woman whose BMI is greater than 35 or is overweight can take twice the amount of time to get pregnant compared to those have a normal BMI and those who have a BMI lower than 19 are underweight might take four times more to vet pregnant. When a woman has excessive body fat, the body will release more estrogen than what the body needs and this can interfere when a woman is ovulating. If a woman tries to lose 5 to 10% of her body weight before trying to get pregnant, she can give her a higher chance of conceiving. Those women who are underweight can stop ovulating or might not be having menstrual periods at all. Another way to help you get pregnant is by taking a prenatal vitamin prior to pregnancy and she needs to find one that is most appropriate for her body and she can maintain it during pregnancy. A woman can also take multivitamins which should contain less than 400 micrograms of folic acid per day. She can also take vitamin B which helps prevent the baby from having defects during birth. Knowing the benefits of folic acid is and taking it in advance is advisable because there is a development of the neural tube into the brain and spine which happens three to four weeks before women find out that they are pregnant.

If you are having problems with your weight, you also need to start eating healthy foods because aside from giving a healthier body, your body will also become more ready to get pregnant. You will have enough supply of nutrients like iron, calcium, and protein. This means that you need to eat vegetables, fruits, whole grains, good fat sources, and protein rich foods. Aside from taking a supplement which has folic acid, green leafy vegetables, cereals, fortified breads, fruits, beans, broccoli, and orange juice also contain vitamin B. When you are trying to conceive, avoid eating too much fish that contain a lot of mercury like king mackerel, tilefish, shark, and swordfish. You also need to reduce your consumption of tuna by 6 ounces every week because it also has a lot of mercury. If you like caffeine, you need to reduce your consumption to only 500 milligrams per day because if you consume more than that, a study shows that it can lead to decrease in fertility. Limit yourself to only 1 to 2 cups of coffee per day which is less than 250 mg has no impact on your chances of getting pregnant. Getting yourself physically active to prepare your body for pregnancy is good, but if you over train your body by frequently doing strenuous workouts can cause interference to your ovulation. Exercising heavily can cause disturbance to your menstrual cycle which means that you have to lessen exercise if you want to get pregnant. You should also not take too much time getting pregnant because as women age, their chances of getting pregnant decreases. As women age, the quantity and quality of the eggs in their ovaries also decrease. A woman's fertility can decline starting the age of 30 and it will decline even more when they reach the age of 37. After the age of 40, it will be extremely hard for women to get pregnant. If you are a heavy smoker, you also need to give up on that regardless if you are a man or a woman because the chemicals nicotine and carbon monoxide found in cigarette smoke can cause problems with fertility. Even secondhand smokers should also stay away from cigarettes. Consuming Marijuana can also cause fertility to decrease. You also need to stop drinking alcohol when trying to get pregnant because she will find it difficult to become pregnant. If a woman is already pregnant, she cannot consume alcohol at all. Your home and workplace should also be fertility-friendly because if you get exposed to too much chemicals found in pesticides, chemical solvents or pollutants that you use at home or in the office, can affect your fertility. You can wear protective clothing, glasses, mask, and gloves to limit your exposure to chemicals that are potentially harmful which is overall not good for your health. Learning how to manage stress is also important because when couples are attempting to get pregnant, they can get stressed. Women should be able to cope with their stress better by finding ways on how they can relax their body and mind. Enough sleep, exercise, and yoga can help a woman cope with stress. You should also know when you need to seek a professional to help you. A couple should have their fertility assessed if the woman is 35 and above and has not gotten pregnant even if they had been having regular sex for the past 6 months without any form of birth control. Women who are more than 35 years old should start seeking help immediately as to why she has not yet become pregnant. If a woman is under 35 and has not become pregnant even after 1 year of unprotected sex should seek help and also her partner.

Chapter 2. Pregnancy Exercises

There are 4 cardiovascular exercises that women can do when they are pregnant. Walking is one way to help pregnant woman. Walking is also a good exercise to do without harming your knees or ankles. This can also be done anywhere and you do not need any other equipment to do it. You can do this during your whole pregnancy. Dancing is also a good cardiovascular exercise because your heart will get pumping and you can dance along with the tunes that you love. You can easily do this at home or you can buy dancing dvds which you can follow. Doing low-impact aerobics will both tone your body and strengthen your heart. Taking classes for women, you will enjoy the company of other pregnant women and you can all share your thoughts together. Swimming is said to be the safest form of exercise for pregnant women because swimming works all of your muscle groups and at the same time providing benefits for your cardiovascular health.

There are 3 flexibility exercises that pregnant women can do to also help in strengthening them. Stretching is great for your body's relaxation and it makes you more limber. It also prevents your muscles from becoming strained. Another exercise you get yourself into is Yoga because it can help keep your muscles be toned, but it is best to mix Yoga with swimming or walking a few times a week to get a full workout. You can also do weight training especially if it has always been a part of your exercise routine, but do not over train yourself because it will also not be good for pregnancy so you must control your amount of weight training to get its benefits for pregnancy.

Chapter 3. Diet Guidelines For Pregnant Women

You need to eat more than one variety of food to get all the nutrients needed by your body. It is recommended that you are eating 6 to 11 servings of breads and grains, then servings of fruit should be 2 to 4 servings, vegetables should be 4 or more servings in a day, the dairy products should be 4 servings, and protein sources should be 3 servings. Fats and sweets are only to be taken sparingly. High-fiber foods like whole grain breads, brown rice, pasta, vegetable, and fruits should also be consumed. Vitamins and minerals will always be an essential part of daily diet especially when a person is pregnant. There are prenatal vitamins that you can take so you are sure that you are getting the amount of vitamins and minerals that you need. You can be advised by your doctor to buy prenatal vitamin over the counter or you can ask your doctor for a prescription. You need to be consuming 4 servings of dairy products per day and foods that are rich in calcium. You need to make sure that the calcium you are getting per day is 1000 to 1300 mg.

When it comes to iron, you should not consume less than 27 mg of it per day. You can get iron from spinach, lean meats, and cereals. During pregnancy you need to have 250 mg of iodine in your body daily because this will help develop the nervous system and brain of your baby. You can get iodine from cottage cheese, milk, cooked navy beans, baked potato, and not more than 8 to 12 ounces of shrimp, cod, and salmon per week. Vitamin C is also very important for pregnant women. Foods like strawberry, orange, grapefruit, papaya, broccoli, tomatoes, green peppers, and Brussel sprouts are good sources of vitamin C. You need to be consuming 70 g of vitamin C per day during pregnancy. You need 0.4 mg of folic acid so you need to eat green leafy vegetables, legumes, and veal to help prevent spina bifida which is a neural tube defect. Eat turnip, squash, cantaloupe, apricots, carrots, sweet potatoes, and beet greens to get vitamin A everyday.

Chapter 4. Herbs That Can Help You Get Pregnant

1 Red Raspberry Leaf – This should primarily be taken when trying to get pregnant, but when you get pregnant, do not consume this herb anymore. Red Raspberry Leaf contains high calcium and if it is combined with herbs especially red clover, it can become highly potent in increasing fertility. This is a leaf that is commonly used to help boost fertility because it is able to tone the uterus, and at the same time strengthen the lining. It is also good for lengthening the luteal phase making it a very conducive environment for pregnancy.

2 Dong Quai – This herb will help in regulating the female hormones and toning the uterus. It helps with the circulation of the blood and helps in purifying it. The properties of this herb are all good for having a healthy reproductive system.

3 Red Clover – This is a rich source of calcium and magnesium to aid in fertility. This herb is very well-known and considered as one of the best to increase women fertility. It will balance the hormone levels and

can help in repairing scars that happen in the fallopian tube so it removes another problem of conception.

4 False Unicorn – This is for vaginal dryness and occurring pains in the ovaries. It is also used for treating infertility that is caused by follicular formations.

5 Black Cohosh – This herb is also very good for the uterus because it helps with the inflammation. It can also be used for painful ovaries to become relieved which can affect the chances of pregnancy.

Chapter 5. When to Test For Pregnancy

You will know that you need to take a pregnancy test if you have missed your period on the first day. If your period is irregular, you will know when to take the pregnancy test. In case you do not know when you will have your period again, you can take a pregnancy test 21 days after you had sex without protection. There are tests that are very sensitive and you can take it days before you have a missed period. Pregnancy tests are done to check the amount of human chorionic gonadotropin (HCG) found in your urine which is a pregnancy hormone. After you get pregnant, your body will produce HCG which happens 2 weeks after you get pregnant. By this time, there will be ample amount of HCG in your urine that can be detected by the test.

The results of the test are mostly correct if it shows positive. If you take a pregnancy test on the first day that you missed your period and it shows positive, this means that you got pregnant 2 weeks ago. If the pregnancy test is showing negative which is a less reliable result, you can choose to take the test again after 1 week if you are not convinced.

Chapter 6. How Age Affects Pregnancy

Age can affect a person's fertility and pregnancy because of the function of the uterus and a woman's health in general as they age. There are a lot of women who aim to have better health by having proper nutrition and exercise so they can get their body ready for pregnancy. Due to age, there is a higher risk of women developing more medical conditions like diabetes, cancer, heart conditions, high blood pressure, and other infections. The uniting chromosomes of the sperm and the egg have a higher risk of leading to miscarriage. There are women who go through pregnancy-induced diabetes if they are older than 35. Age can also affect how the placenta is positioned and can cause premature birth. Due to this, prenatal tests such as amniotic fluid tests and ultrasound and extra care for pregnant women are done more to monitor how their health is progressing.

If parenthood is delayed until after the age of 35, there is an advantage of psychological and social benefits that are often greater than what concerns them physical due to late pregnancy. Women who are at this age have a more prepared mindset in losing a baby due to more experiences compared to younger women who want to get pregnant fast and give birth. Women above 35 have a higher level of maturity when it comes to emotional development and financial capacity to have a child.

Chapter 7. How to Find Out if You Are Ovulating

If you have a change in your cervical fluid, this could mean that you are ovulating. The fluid looks like "egg white" but some women can have cervical fluid that looks different. Ovulation usually happens when there is a lot of wet fluid in the cervix. You can buy products that can help in improving cervical fluid. You should also check your body's basal temperature. That happens in women before they ovulate and it will be noticed that the body's basal temperature is consistent. As the day of the ovulation gets closer, your body's temperature can slightly decline, but you will notice that it will suddenly increase after you have ovulated. The sudden rise in the body temperature is an indication that you have just ovulated. If you track your body's temperature for a few months, you will be able to predict when you are ovulating.

Another way to feel if you are ovulating is if the firmness and ovulation of your cervix starts to change. The cervix will go through a lot of changes while a woman is ovulating. This will make you clearly notice that you are ovulating if your cervix becomes open, soft, high, and wet. Other women take a little time to be able to notice the difference between a cervix that is acting normally and if it is experiencing ovulation.

Chapter 8. How to Deal With a Miscarriage

It is natural that you will feel a little guilty for having a miscarriage, but you need to keep telling yourself that it is not your fault and almost all women who experience miscarriage have no control over what happened. You should not dwell in this guilt and you continue to move on. In case your partner reacts differently with the miscarriage, you do not need to force him to react the same way because people react to situations differently and your partner is probably more of thinking ahead than letting things affect him. You can try conceiving again when you are ready and by being ready means you have undergone physical and emotional factors that were assisted by your OB-GYN and other professionals. Psychologically, there is no definite month when you will be ready. If you think that you will not be able to handle another miscarriage in case it happens again, you need to wait a little more and get the support that you need.

After all of this has happened, you need to learn how to get closure because it will be hard to emotionally move on and you need to stop comparing yourself to others. Everyone deal with a miscarriage differently. You really cannot tell how long you will feel the grief, but you need to just let yourself let go and become ready again for pregnancy. You cannot keep blaming yourself because of what you have gone through. These things happen and you have no control over it.

Conclusion

When you are trying to get pregnant, being healthy is number one because it will all lead to complications of you do not start with this one. Your body needs to be healthy enough to be ready for pregnancy and strong enough to handle being pregnant. Make sure that you are following the proper diet that your baby needs and stay away from alcohol. All of this boils down to good habits and healthy practices. Giving birth to a healthy baby is the best thing that can happen to any mother because carrying a baby for 9 months in your womb is not that easy and your body goes through changes that may sometimes surprise you. As a mother, it is your responsibility to keep your child healthy from the time that he or she is in your womb until they grow up. A baby's strong body will start from the nutrients that you take while you are still pregnant because these nutrients help in making your child's immune system healthy and strong to not be prone to sickness and infection. You need to also be prepared for having a child because your child will need all the support he or she can get from you.

Being a responsible mom means that you are willing to make sacrifices for your child. Keep yourself healthy, strong, and emotionally ready in raising a child because a child will be one of the greatest gifts you will ever receive. A healthy child will also lead to less worries and you will also become very happy as parent.

Thank You Page

I want to personally thank you for reading my book. I hope you found information in this book useful and I would be very grateful if you could leave your honest review about this book. I certainly want to thank you in advance for doing this.

If you have the time, you can check my other books too.

www.ingramcontent.com/pod-product-compliance
Lightning Source LLC
LaVergne TN
LVHW021748060526
838200LV00052B/3538